ADHD Symptom and Strategies

BY JEFFREY POWELL

The Ultimate Guide for Understanding and Handling Attention Deficit Disorder in Adults and Children

2nd Edition

Table of Contents

Introduction

I want to thank you and congratulate you for purchasing the book, "ADHD Symptoms and Strategies: The Ultimate Guide for Understanding and Handling Attention Deficit Disorder in Adults and Children".

This book contains proven steps and strategies on how to deal with a child or adult suffering from ADHD. This condition not only affects the person; it also affects relationships with family members as well as performance in school and in the workplace. It can also negatively affect the sufferer's self-esteem. While this condition has no cure, it can be positively and effectively dealt with.

Read on to find out how to live a better and more meaningful life despite ADHD.

Thanks again for purchasing this book, I hope you enjoy it!

Chapter 1 Digging for the Truth: Myths and Facts about ADHD

Everyone has probably heard about Attention Deficit Hyperactivity Disorder or ADHD. But does everyone really understand what this condition entails? Unfortunately, only a few really do. As a matter of fact, like other disorders, ADHD is surrounded by myths and misconceptions. These misunderstandings create stereotypes. And most even question the degree of seriousness of ADHD.

The purpose of this chapter is to cut to the chase and straighten these misconceptions out once and for all. So without further delay, below are the most common myths and misconceptions about ADHD and the truth behind them.

ADHD is not really a disorder.

Some people may think it is made up like other mental disorders. It can be difficult to understand something that does not affect you or those around you. But just because this thing is unfamiliar does not make it less real.

ADHD is a mental disorder. It comes with a biological component. In fact, it could be inherited. One study about ADHD revealed that diagnosed children possess gene variations that other children do not have. And these variations go by the hundreds.

Only children have ADHD.

The common belief is ADHD like other childlike traits can be outgrown. But the reality of it is that children with ADHD grow up and continue to struggle. It is important to note however, that as a child with ADHD grows, the symptoms may seem different.

Hyperactivity is a common symptom in children. But as these children grow, hyperactivity tends to subside or at least diminish. Inattentive symptoms, however, continue to exist. In fact, it can possibly worsen. There is much to be expected from adults and when they fail to manage those expectations. In which case, the symptoms can become disabling.

Adults with ADHD may still feel an "itch." The tendency to be on the move and be active can still be quite strong. Inside, they cannot help but be restless. So, in truth, both children and adults are affected by this mental disorder.

Adults with ADHD are hyperactive.

Hyperactivity may be the most visible symptom of ADHD but it does not apply to all. As mentioned previously, children with hyperactive symptoms experience diminished hyperactivity by the time they reach adolescence and it can extend up to their adult years. Again, it is important to emphasize that some people with ADHD don't even have hyperactive symptoms to begin with.

While some ADHD patients are hyperactive, others are the inattentive type. They may not be hyperactive but they suffer from distractibility and disorganization. They may also struggle with poor time management and forgetfulness.

Children with ADHD should not be treated with stimulant medication as such may lead to addiction.

This could be a parent's worst nightmare. And this misconception makes most hesitant to allow their children to be administered with stimulant medication. It is enough their children struggles with ADHD. They do not need an addiction problem too.

The concern of parents is perfectly understandable. But it is important to note that there is no actual indication that stimulant medication can cause addiction. In fact, stimulants can significantly help reduce the debilitating symptoms of ADHD. Individuals who are under stimulant medication even demonstrate lower risks to substance abuse as compared to those who do not take the said medication.

Proponents of this myth use animal studies to support their claim. Although it is true that stimulant medication in animals causes sensitization which means they show drug seeking behavior, they forget to mention the dosage used in these studies. These animals are administered with as much as 50 to 200 times more than the dose used for people with ADHD.

With the right dosage, stimulant medication can actually help children in their social and academic functioning. And as a result, they experience a boost in self esteem and are less likely to self medicate into their adulthood. That translates to lower risk of substance abuse in the future. In fact, earlier treatment reduces substance abuse tendencies. This is according to a study conducted by researchers from Harvard Medical School.

ADHD is not that special. It is more likely that everyone at this day and age suffers from ADHD.

We live in chaos. The technology driven world we live in makes us feel overwhelmed and distracted. It is quite easy for us to get sidetracked. With so many distractions around us, we become forgetful. We find it much more difficult to focus. But it does not necessarily mean we have ADHD. What sets people with ADHD apart from the rest of the population is that their moments of distraction are higher.

Individuals with ADHD are simply lacking in motivation which is why they won't focus and fail to complete tasks.

For most people, focusing and working on tasks to completion is a matter of honing their desire and fueling their drive for accomplishment. But for people with ADHD, it is actually a matter of ability. They do want to complete what they have started. But they simply cannot. If you ask a friend with ADHD to drop by the grocery store and pick up something and they fail to. It is not that they are lazy. It is that they simply forget.

ADHD people disregard consequences.

Whether or not people with ADHD are mindful about consequences is not the issue. The real problem has to do with their ability to process the concept of consequences. They are aware of the fact that something must be done in a certain way. However, it is tough for them to make it stick to their brains.

ADHD is not a big deal.

It is typical for people with ADHD to struggle in all aspects of their lives. They experience problems in big responsibilities including handling jobs. They even struggle with simple tasks such as paying the bills before its due. ADHD is especially tough on relationships.

One study shows that low credit scores is not the only thing common about individuals with ADHD. They also tend to have much higher cholesterol levels. And this comes from the fact that they have extreme difficulty in handling a wide range of matters with regard to their lifestyle.

If you have ADHD, you simply need to try harder.

This mental disorder truly lays down plenty of obstacles. And it takes effort to overcome such obstacles. Effort however, is merely not enough. How can you force a person with poor eyesight to try harder so he can see well?

It is not that individuals with ADHD do not try hard. They in fact, have to try hard for a lifetime. The problem is there is no proof of their efforts. And for this reason, it is crucial to deal with ADHD using appropriate treatment and strategies that are ADHD-friendly. And that means taking into account how a person's brain with ADHD processes information.

Ritalin can cure ADHD.

Psychostimulant medication is commonly used for the treatment of ADHD. And Ritalin is one of these medications. It actually helps especially with children to become less hyperactive and be more focused. However, for Ritalin to be at its most effective, it should be used only as a part of a bigger treatment plan. And every treatment plan must also include academic help because that is crucial in behavior-modification.

ADHD is merely a result of bad parenting.

Kids with ADHD are simply out of control. And their parents are to blame for their misbehavior. All these kids need discipline. That is how a lot of people think. But that is not true.

Again, ADHD is a real disorder. Some people do not seem to understand that the brains of people with ADHD are wired differently and that makes it difficult for them to control their behavior. The brain activity and brain size of kids with ADHD are distinctively different. They may make inappropriate comments and they may constantly fidget. These signs do not make them "bad kids" or of "bad parenting." Rather, these are signs of their medical condition.

ADHD is common among boys and not on girls.

Most children and adults are male. Boys are two times more likely to be diagnosed of ADHD. But that does not mean girls and women do not suffer from the same disorder. The truth is the symptoms of ADHD may just be overlooked among girls and this could be the reason why most girls remain undiagnosed. Issues with attention and misbehavior do happen in both boys and girls. But girls are less likely to cause a commotion in class.

Ritalin may affect a child's growth.

Ritalin has proven to be an effective treatment for ADHD. But aside from the misconception that stimulant medication increases addiction tendencies, there is also a misunderstanding about the medication's effect on a child's growth. Although it is possible that Ritalin affects growth in children, studies do prove that such effect, if any, is nothing more but temporary. As a matter of fact, children who take Ritalin throughout adolescence do grow to normal height.

Alternative treatment could cure ADHD.

There are plenty of advertised miracle cures for all sorts of medical conditions. And it seems some people buy into the claim. For ADHD, herbs and vitamins including alternative techniques are believed to cure ADHD once and for all. However, these so called "miracle cures" are baseless. There are no scientific studies to back up their claims.

Some of these "cures" include mineral supplements and megavitamins, Candida treatment, applied kinesiology and medication for motion sickness among others.

Too much sugar causes ADHD in children.

Sugar rush may cause hyperactivity. It is wrong however, to conclude that sugar causes ADHD. There are no research studies to prove high sugar dose affects a child's brain size.

ADHD does not coexist with other conditions.

The truth is ADHD is associated with other conditions including mood, anxiety and conduct disorders as well as learning disabilities. Most children who are diagnosed with ADHD have been found to suffer from another condition.

When ADHD coexists with conduct disorder as seen in 35 percent of children diagnosed of ADHD, the child is more likely to demonstrate hostile and defiant behavior. This child can lose his temper easily.

25 percent of kids with ADHD also suffer from anxiety disorders. 18 percent of them have mood disorders too. And while ADHD is not considered a learning disability, the disorder makes it tougher for children to acquire specific skills. The child is more likely to do poorly in math or reading. This is why school is tough for children with ADHD.

A child with ADHD is hopeless.

If your child is diagnosed with ADHD, you should never lose hope. Having the disorder does not mean he will not amount to anything. Many people with ADHD have been successful in their chosen field. Some of them grew up to be politicians, scientists and famous artists including Elvis Presley, Robin Williams, Vincent Van Gogh, Wright Brothers, Frank Lloyd Wright, Benjamin Franklin, JFK, Mozart and Abraham Lincoln among many others.

What you need to understand is that people with ADHD needs all the support they can get. And early diagnosis and treatment is their key to success. Although it may be difficult to understand, a person with ADHD can get all the support he needs no matter how uninterested or uncooperative this person may seem to be.

Chapter 2 Understanding ADHD

ADHD- Attention deficit hyperactivity disorder- is one of the childhood disorders becoming more and more common in recent years. This is a neurobehavioral disorder, which starts to develop during childhood and may persist into adulthood. The defining characteristic of ADHD is difficulty keeping focus and attention, hyperactivity and difficulty in controlling the different behaviors.

Factors that cause ADHD

Years of studying ADHD has not yet yielded a definite cause. There are factors, though, that are linked to its development.

Genes

One of the factors found to play a major role in ADHD is genes. Studies showed that ADHD has a large tendency to run in families. Children that have ADHD were found to carry a certain gene that causes brain tissues to be thinner than normal. The thin tissues are more often found in the areas of the brain associated with attention. As the children who have this gene grew up, the brain tissue matured with the normal thickness, and the symptoms of ADHD consequently improved.

Other factors

Aside from genes that play a major role in ADHD development, other factors have some role. Although, these factors do not automatically and significantly cause ADHD when present alone.

Environmental factors

Exposure to certain toxins in the environment has been found potentially linked to the development of ADHD. Chemicals include cigarette smoke and alcohol exposure while in uterus has been found to possibly cause ADHD in the baby later in life. Preschoolers exposed to high levels of lead in preschools may also increase the risk for ADHD.

Brain injuries

Trauma to the brain may cause changes in the structure and function of the brain tissues, which may lead to symptoms of ADHD. However, among children diagnosed with ADHD, a very small percentage has history of traumatic brain injury.

Sugar

A popular idea about ADHD is the link of early exposure to refined sugars to the development of ADHD. The idea is that children who ate foods that contain refined sugars are at higher risk for ADHD. The symptoms of those who already have ADHD worsen with it.

Studies done related to this idea discount the claim. One study even found that mothers who thought their children were given aspartame, a sugar substitute more commonly known as Nutrasweet, were more critical of their children's behavior and rated them as more hyperactive. Further studies need to confirm if there is really a significant effect of refined sugars to ADHD.

Food additives

Unlike the case of refined sugars, studies about the link between food additives and ADHD show possible relationship. Artificial colors and preservatives can increase activity, which can trigger the hyperactive state of ADHD symptoms.

The Signs and Symptoms of ADHD

The key behaviors that define ADHD are hyperactivity, inattention and impulsivity. These are all normal behaviors in children. However, in those suffering from ADHD, these occur more often and more pronounced than what is considered as normal behavior. In order to diagnose a child, he must be exhibiting the symptoms for more than 6 months, more often and more severe than other children of the same age.

Inattention symptoms include any of the following behaviors:

- The child is easily distracted when performing certain tasks, switching from one task to another, without completing any. The child misses details and forgets things more often than what is normally observed in other children of the same age.

- The child has difficulty focusing on a single task or activity.

- The child easily becomes bored after a few minutes into an activity, unless it is something that the child enjoys.

- The child has difficulty in focusing his attention on

things like learning something new, and in organizing and completing tasks.

- The child has frequent trouble in completing or submitting homework on time. He also often loses things needed for the completion of certain task and activities like pencils, erasers and toys.

- The child does not seem to listen when being spoken to.

- The child is often observed daydreaming, moving slowly when going about the activity and becomes easily confused.

- The child has difficulty understanding information quickly and accurately as other children do.

- The child can be observed struggling when following instructions.

Hyperactivity symptoms in ADHD include the following behaviors:

- The child fidgets and squirms in his seat more frequently than others do.

- The child is very talkative, telling stories nonstop.

- The child dashes around the room. He touches, handles and plays with everything in sight.

- The child has trouble sitting still for certain activities like story time, eating meals or during school.

- The child is constantly moving around.

- The child has difficulty engaging in quiet activities or tasks.

Symptoms of impulsivity in ADHD include behaviors like:

- The child is very impatient.

- The child is often observed blurting out inappropriate comments even in the company of strangers. He shows emotions without any evident restraint. H acts without any consideration for the consequences that the actions may bring.

- The child has difficulty waiting for turns or for anything they want.

- The child often interrupts conversations or activities of others.

Subtypes

Some people affected with ADHD manifest all three main symptoms of impulsivity (difficulty exercising control over behaviors), inattention and hyperactivity. One or more of these behaviors may become more dominant than others are, and are the basis for the subtypes of ADHD. The symptoms should also be observed for the last 6 months, in the least.

Predominantly hyperactive-impulsive

A predominantly hyperactive-impulsive ADHD type manifests the following:

- There are more symptoms observed under the hyperactivity and impulsivity categories. The observed symptoms should be six or more.

- Symptoms under the inattention category are still observed, but to a lesser degree, frequency and number.

Predominantly inattentive

A person with a predominantly inattentive subtype exhibits the following:

- Majority of the observed symptoms belong under the inattentive category, with at least 6 symptoms noted.

- Symptoms under the hyperactivity and impulsivity categories are also present but are less than 6 symptoms, and are less in severity and frequency.

- Those suffering from ADHD of this subtype often sit quietly but do not pay attention to what they are doing. They are often overlooked as having ADHD.

- Those under this subtype are also less likely to be observed acting out or having difficulties in getting along with others.

Combined hyperactive-impulsive and inattentive

Under this category, the following behaviors are notable:

- There are at least 6 symptoms observed that are classified under the inattention category and at least 6 under the hyperactivity-impulsivity category.

- This subcategory is more commonly observed among ADHD sufferers.

A lot of parents and teachers miss recognizing the symptoms of ADHD, especially those with symptoms under the inattention category. These children often are able to work quietly and seldom act out. They are also able to get along with other children. Because they are not as disruptive, these children are often left alone. They seem to be able to work independently but in reality, they are not paying any attention at all to the task. Hyperactivity-impulsivity symptoms may also be missed. Parents and teachers may treat the symptoms as emotional or disciplinary problems, and not as ADHD.

Who are at risk for developing ADHD

This condition is one of the most common childhood disorders. The average onset of ADHD is 7 years old, occurring four times more among males than among females. The symptoms may even persist until adolescence and adulthood. Adolescent and adult ADHD are likely from an undiagnosed childhood ADHD or inadequately treated one. The number of children between the ages of 4 and 17 diagnosed with this disorder are increasing in recent years. In 2011, about 11% of this age group suffers from ADHD.

ADHD and Other Mental Health Problems

ADHD is commonly accompanied by other mental health issues. Treatment for each patient may vary significantly because of the presence of such mental health problems. Below is a list of the most common disorders linked with ADHD.

- Anxiety and Depression

  People both children and adults who have ADHD, may also suffer from anxiety and depression. When these problems are resolved with treatment, the patient can cope with ADHD in a more effective manner. At the same time, as ADHD is properly and adequately treated, the patient's anxiety and depression may also be reduced. In which case, a comprehensive type of and appropriate treatment is necessary.

- Bipolar Disorder

Distinguishing between ADHD and bipolar symptoms can be a challenge because they often share similar symptoms. Bipolar disorder is characterized by extreme moods that usually occur in a spectrum. It can start with a debilitating depression and shift to uncontrollable mania. In between these two extreme states, the patient may be able to experience normal moods.

Children with bipolar disorder however, are much more different. Their extreme mood swings can happen within an hour. There are instances when the child may experience depression and mania at the same time.

A patient with both ADHD and bipolar disorder often have reduced sleep needs and unbelievably high energy levels.

- Conduct Disorder

This is considered to be a more serious type of antisocial behavior. It can occur in 20 to 40 percent of patients with ADHD. Someone who has conduct disorder violates social norms and disregards the rights of others. Physical aggression, bullying, cruelty

21

to animals, lying, destruction of property, truancy, stealing, vandalism, and over-aggressive behavior are among the symptoms of this disorder. Someone suffers from ADHD and conduct disorder at the same time are at a higher risk of getting in trouble with the authorities. And they are also more likely to experiment with drugs.

- Learning Disability

  There are about 20 to 30 percent of kids with ADHD who also have a learning disability. Children with this problem often have difficulty reading and spelling. However, when a child received appropriate treatment, he can learn more adequately and successfully.

- Oppositional Defiant Disorder

  This disorder is characterized by hostility, disobedience and defiance. And it occurs in more than 50 percent of children with ADHD. It is more likely to occur in boys too.

  Children with both disorders may easily lose their temper, disobey rules and argue with adults. They are more likely to annoy other people in a deliberate manner. They may blame others for the mistakes they commit. They may feel spiteful and resentful as well.

These facts should not serve to scare or worry you more. It is important that you become aware. With understanding come better solutions. And for this reason, subjecting your child, a loved one or yourself to ADHD assessment is crucial.

Chapter 3 Diagnosing ADHD in Children

Perhaps you are worried about your child. You have read about the ADHD symptoms and you feel like your child fits the bill. But how can you really tell when what troubles your child troubles other kids too? How do you know it is something to worry about? When do you take a step into finding out whether or not your child has ADHD?

The simple answer to these questions is to simply listen to what your gut tells you. When you feel that things are not right with your child's behavior and if you feel it makes him incredibly unhappy, perhaps you should start finding a doctor to help you. If these behavioral issues start affecting your family, interfering with school then you should know it must be tougher for your kid. When you feel it is the right thing to do, set up an appointment.

The good news is early intervention coupled with proper treatment help with better results. And that could mean a whole lot for your child's future.

What to Expect from ADHD Evaluation

Before a doctor can conclude a case of ADHD, he requires plenty of information. And such information is gathered with the help of clinical interviews. There are behavior checklists and questionnaires that must be completed. This will allow the medical professional to assess problematic behaviors. Potentially, further evaluations may be required in the form of observation including educational and psychological testing.

If a child is under evaluation, the cooperation of both parents and teachers is crucial including other adults that can help shed light on the child's behavior provided different settings. This may include a thorough interview with the adults concerned. In addition, complete physical examination is also necessary in order to identify other possible medical conditions that may be causing the problematic behaviors. In which case, the medical professional may need to refer to a family medical history.

How to Help Prepare Your Child for ADHD Evaluation

There are various stages for the evaluation. Understand that while this must be difficult for you, it can be tougher for the child. With this said, below is a list of suggestions for preparation and other things you should expect.

Before Your Initial Appointment

When you request an appointment for evaluation, you are more likely to receive some questionnaires and checklist about your child's behavior. You are expected to complete all these forms before you meet with the doctor.

The forms help the medical professional learn some information about your family and the child concerned. They may also include medical history. You may also find questions that pertain to the behavioral and developmental history of your child.

In addition to the filled out forms, you must also prepare copies of psychological and school records. If your child has undergone evaluations previously, copies of the said testing will be helpful, too. The doctor will be as detailed as possible.

It is important you are well prepared for the documents as well as the questions he may ask of you.

Parent Interview

When a child is concerned, ADHD testing requires a parent interview. In fact, it comprises a major part of the evaluation. To prepare for the process, you can create a list or jot down notes about any specific concern you may have with regard to your child. Being thorough is important. Note of where and when such problems occur whether in school, at home or around the neighborhood. Does your child's problematic behavior happen when he is with his peers or during after-school activities? Determine when such problems occur more often with your child than any other kids his age. Is it typical or could it be something else.

It will be helpful to have a chat with your child's teachers too. Ask about their concerns, if any. Expect the doctor to hand out behavior checklists to your child's school mentors as well.

Aside from ongoing concerns, it will help a lot for you to recall other problems in the past that may relate with your child's troubles now. When did all these problems begin and how long has it been going on? Because the medical professional will need the child's medical history, the pediatrician may be contacted as well. Write down everything you remember that may be relevant. Share the details no matter how trivial they may seem to you.

If there are any issues within your family that may have a huge impact on your child, you should bring them up too. Think of any losses or changes that have occurred. It may affect your child more than you know. Was there death or a serious health problem affecting one of the family members? Did you recently moved or did your child changed school? These are issues that are quite sensitive. And it is understandable for you to face difficulty discussing them but as it is important in a proper evaluation and accurate diagnosis, you should take a step forward and do it for the sake of your child.

With a list of pertinent information on your hands, you will be better prepared for the doctor's questions. And to make sure the doctor gets a good idea of how your child is like, write down your kid's strengths as well. If appointments and testing have been conducted before, bring copies of the report. Write down names of people who may be helpful including their corresponding contact information.

Child Interview

In addition to the parent interview, it is also essential for the doctor to meet the child. The doctor may assess or measure your child's understanding about why you have taken him there. The child's perceptions will be gauged too. But the main purpose of the interview is to assess the developmental and behavioral skills of the child.

When faced with something or someone unfamiliar, children often behave differently. Rest assured that the medical professional is trained and aware of this. If the doctor determines the possibility of a learning disability or any trace of developmental or emotional issue, he may request further educational evaluation as well as psychological testing.

Other tests that may be necessary include neuro-developmental screening and physical examination from a pediatrician to rule out the possibility of medical conditions leading to the ADHD-like symptoms. In some cases, the doctors also request for language and formal speech assessments. Overall, the evaluation for ADHD may take a minimum of two or three hours.

Talking about ADHD with Your Child

After diagnosis, what then? How do you exactly tell your child he has ADHD? You may be afraid your child will be labeled. And as a parent, you feel protective. Understand however, that knowing the truth about the diagnosis can even be a relief to your child. It explains why he's been struggling. And this knowledge will grant him a sense of control.

What do you think is harder to take? Is it being called "stupid" or knowing you have ADHD and that is what makes you different? When you talk to your child about the diagnosis, the mystery behind his being different is unveiled. What he needs to do or go through in order to get better becomes clearer. In other words, explaining ADHD to your child has a positive impact. And try to focus on this.

So where do you begin? Below is a list of suggestions.

Ask help from your doctor.

After the assessment when the results are in, the doctor will more likely to talk to you first and explain the diagnosis. Understandably, this can be a learning process. Then, it becomes your responsibility to explain it to your child. But that does not mean you cannot ask help from an expert. If you do not exactly know much yet about ADHD, you can ask the doctor to back you up in case your child has questions. The doctor is in the proper place to provide pieces of information that are as accurate as possible. It will help with you as well as your child's understanding of ADHD.

Choose the right approach.

You have to be mindful about your approach too. It is important that you stay positive. This could be hard for you too. But it is essential that you stay strong for your child. He needs to know he can count on you to hold him steady. Try to learn as much as you can about the disorder first. This way, you'd be more comfortable discussing it with him.

Talk to him in his language. But at the same time, you have to maintain a matter-of-fact way of saying it. You have now become aware of the reason for his troubles, his inattention and all the problems he's been having. So you are now in a much better position to address the issues in a more effective manner.

Encourage your child to ask questions. And do not worry if you do not know the answer yet. Reassure him that everything is going to be alright. And together, as a family, you will work things out. Learn together and work together.

Determine your child's strengths and help him address his weaknesses.

We all have our own set of strengths and weaknesses. And your child probably has to. Help your child by determining his areas of interest. Build on his strengths. At the same time, help him figure out a way to minimize his difficulties. Let him know you are there for him a hundred percent.

Read books together.

Books about ADHD will not only be helpful to your child. It is also helpful to you and the rest of your family. You can read it to him or if he is old enough, he can read it himself. Make sure you give him space to digest the information.

Suggest positive role models.

ADHD may be an obstacle but there are ways around it. ADHD should not stand in the way of your child's future and his success as an individual. To help foster a positive outlook, suggest role models. Perhaps there is someone close to you who has ADHD who your child looks up to. Otherwise, there are writers, artists, business entrepreneurs, doctors, athletes and other successful people who happen to have ADHD too. It is important you help your child understand that the disorder does not make him. Rather, it is a small part of him. And it makes him wonderful all the more.

Chapter 4 Diagnosing ADHD in Adults

Many people consider ADHD as a disorder that only occurs in childhood. This stems from the misconception that ADHD is something that can be outgrown into adulthood. But the reality of it is it can go beyond teenage years. It can last a lifetime. And the problematic symptoms that come with it can be experienced from childhood to adolescence to adulthood.

Children with ADHD under hyperactive-impulsive type demonstrate physical hyperactivity but such diminishes with age. However the subtle symptoms in childhood including distractibility, inattention, restlessness, disorganization, poor self-regulation and planning, verbal impulsiveness and forgetfulness often continue or worsen to the point of impairing an adult's life most especially when ADHD is left untreated.

When is the right time to get screened for ADHD?

What if there is someone you know who may have ADHD? How do you get help for this person? What if you feel like you may have ADHD?

The first step is diagnosis. And like with kids, the key here is gut feeling. If your life or that of the person you know is compromised because of disorganization, lack of planning, forgetfulness and other troubles then go ahead and set up an ADHD screening. A person who is untreated for a long time can experience chronic problems. For this person, life is stressful and incredibly overwhelming. The quality of life can be improved. And it shall start with getting diagnosed correctly.

Like with children, there is a lot of information the doctor requires to correctly arrive at a diagnosis. For instance, the entire childhood history must be reviewed. The doctor also needs to assess any existing evidence of impairment. Alternative causes of ADHD-like symptoms must also be evaluated along with other considerations.

Revisiting Childhood History

ADHD usually occurs on childhood and it is carried on to adulthood. If an adult gets screened for ADHD, the doctor will have to revisit his childhood history in search of the presence of ADHD symptoms. This is crucial in meeting the set criteria for diagnosis.

This means although the patient was not diagnosed of ADHD as a child, the symptoms could have already been present then. Such symptoms may include lack of self control and inattention especially between the crucial stages of development from 12 to 14 years old. In other cases of ADHD, symptoms may not have been present during childhood but a medical condition or brain injury may also bring about the same symptoms.

Evidence of Impairment

Is there significant impairment or deficit experienced by the adult regarding functioning? Do such problems occur across settings? Are the issues affecting this adult's relationships, work or family and social life? An adult with ADHD means that this person experiences struggles and impairment on his daily life. The criteria for ADHD diagnosis does not just take into account the pervasiveness of the problem. It is important that the impulsive and inattentive symptoms are also chronic.

Identifying Alternative Causes

The presenting ADHD symptoms may be caused by another medical condition. The doctor must determine the possibility of other explanations. Everything else must be ruled out first and the doctor must perform all the assessments and tests necessary. This is crucial in reaching an accurate diagnosis.

Other Considerations

In addition to ADHD, the doctor is also responsible for identifying other conditions the patient may be suffering from. For instance, in adults, ADHD may come with depression and anxiety. For those who have not been diagnosed and never gone ADHD treatment before, substance abuse is also a possibility. This is important in determining the most appropriate approach and the most effective treatment plan.

What happens during the evaluation?

ADHD evaluation for adults may last for about three hours. The assessment includes a thorough interview with the patient, the spouse or partner as well as with the siblings and parent of the patient. This is referred to as clinical interview and the questions are designed to assess the medical, developmental, social, school and work history of the patient. This also provides hints about the patient's childhood history and sheds light to any relevant behavioral problems he may already have back then.

For the patient, rating scales, questionnaires and intellectual screenings are also conducted. The doctor will use certain measures to assess the level of distractibility and sustained attention. If applicable, the doctor will also conduct further tests to determine any learning disabilities.

Medical history from childhood to present is important. It will help in ruling out any medical conditions that may lead to the problems. Psychological testing is part of a more comprehensive assessment and it can support findings from previous testing.

How to talk about it?

It may be tougher to talk to a child about ADHD. But talking with an adult does not make it any easier either. The only advantage is that an adult may be in a better position to understand what is going on.

What's important is to keep positive about it. Be realistic but not hopeless. Talk in a matter-of-fact way but not heartless. Whether it is your friend, your spouse, your sibling or anyone else, you have to be supportive as much as you can. And more importantly, you have to be patient.

Chapter 5 Treatment Options

Contrary to what other people think, there is no actual cure for ADHD. Treatments for ADHD aim at controlling the symptoms to improve the social functioning. With the right treatments, the person with ADHD is able to succeed in school and grow up to live productive lives. More researches are conducted in search for more effective treatments and management of the symptoms, to allow the individual to live a better life. New tools are also being used in order gain a better understanding of ADHD that would help in finding more ways for effective treatment and possible prevention.

Treatments for ADHD include medications to control symptoms, psychotherapy to exercise more control over behavioral symptoms and improve social functioning, special education to cater to the symptoms and trainings to help in leading a more productive life.

Medications

Medications given to ADHD are not designed to cure the disorder. They are given in order to control the symptoms. They are only effective as long as the drug is taken. These medications help in keeping attention in order to complete tasks such as schoolwork. The dosage is adjusted all throughout the treatment, depending on the response to the medication and to the needs.

Stimulants are the most common prescribed medication to treat symptoms of ADHD. It may seem odd to give stimulants to a hyperactive or impulsive person, but the effect of this type of drug is opposite in ADHD. They have a calming effect. They reduce impulsivity and hyperactivity, and improve attention abilities in order to help maintain focus on learning and in completing tasks. In some patients, these medications are able to improve physical coordination.

The response to medications differs among those with ADHD. A certain drug at a certain dosage may work for one but not for all. Side effects also vary among those taking the various medications. More often than not, people who suffer from ADHD may need to try several medications before a suitable drug is found. Close monitoring is necessary while under drug treatments.

Stimulant medications are available in various forms such as liquid medicine preparations, capsule, pills or skin patch. They may also be short acting, long acting or in an extended-release varieties. The active ingredients in these varieties are the same but the time of release varies. Short-acting drugs need to be taken at several times a day compared to long-acting ones. Extended-release forms are those that can be taken at least once a day, but are more prone to side effects and over dosage. The key to finding what works is through close monitoring and coordinating with a physician, other health workers, parents and teachers.

Side effects

Stimulants can cause some side effects, most of which are minor that usually disappear over time or if the dosage is lowered. Some of the common side effects are:

- Decreased appetite

  Aside from the calming effect of stimulants in ADHD, they may also depress the appetite. To avoid complications like malnutrition, make sure to give healthy meals. Monitor the child's growth and weight gain. Work closely with a nutritionist to adequately provide for the child's growing up needs.

- Sleep disturbances

Stimulants may cause difficulty sleeping. Report this to the doctor so that some adjustments can be made to reduce sleep problems. The dosage may be lowered, or a short-acting form be prescribed. The medications can be taken at a much earlier time. Medications scheduled for afternoons or evenings may also be stopped. Sometimes, antidepressants in low doses may be prescribed.

Aside from medications, sleep problems may be addressed by promoting a relaxing and restful environment. Remove any distracting items in the room like toys and television. Provide soft music that will lull the child to sleep. Dim light can also decrease stimulation and promote sleep. Warm milk before bedtime can promote relaxation and improve the quality of sleep.

- Reportable side effects

Although less common, some side effects may appear that require reporting to a physician. Tics, which are sudden, involuntary and repetitive sounds or movements may appear. Report this to a physician, as dosage adjustment may cause tics to go away. Personality changes, like suddenly becoming unemotional or flat should be reported to the doctor because this may be an adverse effect of the drug.

Stimulants are safe to use in children as long as proper dosage, administration and monitoring are observed. There is also very little evidence that stimulant use can cause substance dependence or abuse.

- Other side effects include headaches (may go away after some time), upset stomach (relieved when drug is taken with food) and increased blood pressure (change positions slowly).

Contraindications

While stimulants have been seen to reduce symptoms in 70% of adults and 70-80% of children, some conditions contraindicate its use.

- People with glaucoma are not to take stimulants. In glaucoma, the pressure inside the eyes is high. When stimulants are taken, the pupils constrict, which worsens pressure buildup within the eyes. This situation can lead to blindness.

- People with severe anxiety, nervousness, agitation and tension will have worsening symptoms if taking stimulants.

- Those taking MAOIs or monoamine oxidase inhibitors (antidepressants) may have adverse side effects when taken with stimulants.

- Motor tics or a family history of Tourette's syndrome may be triggered or worsen with stimulants.

- Psychotic history (personal or family) can resurface when stimulants are taken for ADHD.

Directions for use

The following guidelines are followed to assure safety and effectiveness of stimulant medication therapy:

- Follow the dosage and schedules strictly.

- Start stimulant medication therapy during the weekends to see how the child would react to the medication. Weekends are best so that no important schoolwork or activity will be compromised. Also, the parent is likely to be more available to be with the child.

- Medications are started at a low dose and gradually increased until the symptoms are effectively controlled.

- Medications are given at a regular schedule. Inform the child's teachers, school nurses or other caregivers to delegate the administration of medication, especially if the parent cannot be with the child for an entire day.

- Medication vacations or holidays may be planned if the response is good, and if activities permit going on a medication-free day or days.

- In case medications are missed, do not double the dose. Continue with the next scheduled dose, as if no schedule is missed. Never ever catch up by doubling or giving additional doses.

Sample Drugs

- Methylphenidate

  This is the most common drug given to ADHD. It includes brand names like Ritalin, Concerta and Metadate. These are all taken orally, and act on the brain as a psychostimulant.

  Daytrana is a skin patch form of medication to treat ADHD. One patch is applied on the hip area, every day. Each patch delivers the drug methylphenidate over a 9-hour period.

- Dexmethylphenidate (Focalin)

  This drug increases the dopamine levels in the body. dopamine is a natural neurotransmitter that plays a major role in cognitive functions like focus and attention.

- Strattera

  This is the only FDA-approved non-stimulant drug for ADHD treatment. The generic name of Strattera is atomoxitine. This drug helps control ADHD symptoms by increasing the levels of norepinephrine in the body.

  The drug works longer than stimulant drugs, the effects lasts for more than 24 hours. Hence, there is less frequency of administration, suitable for those who cannot give frequent doses at regular times. However, the downside of Strattera is that it is not as effective as stimulant drugs in controlling hyperactivity symptoms.

Side effects of Strattera include:

- Headaches
- Dizziness
- Sleepiness
- Mood swings
- Nausea and vomiting
- Upset stomach
- Abdominal pain

Psychotherapy

Psychotherapy is a treatment option that targets behavioral and social aspects of ADHD. Behavioral therapy is a type of psychotherapy given as part of ADHD treatment. The goal is to help the child change the undesirable behavior. It includes providing practical assistance when performing tasks like schoolwork or when working through emotional difficulties. This type of psychotherapy involves teaching the child about monitoring own behavior, recognizing the behavioral symptoms of ADHD and learning to control them. The approach includes giving self-praise or rewards for acting according to expected norms. Anger management and thinking before acting or saying something is one concrete example. To help the child to be able to organize and complete tasks, provide chore lists. Set clear rules that the child should follow. Structured routines are also of great help.

Social skills are also taught through psychotherapy. Skills like how to wait for turns, sharing, responding to teasing, reading facial expressions and recognizing the tone of voice, and how to respond appropriately to these situations are just some the things taught in psychotherapy.

Treating Adults with ADHD

Adolescents and adults can have ADHD, too. It may stem from an undiagnosed childhood ADHD that became evident during the older years or an ADHD that failed to improve with maturing years. The same treatment options are available, with some adjustments to match the developmental level of the ADHD sufferer.

- Medications

    Antidepressants are more often used to treat or control ADHD symptoms in adults. Tricyclic antidepressants, in particular, are used to influence the levels of norepinephrine and dopamine in the body.

    New studies show that venlafaxine (Effexor) is effective in boosting norepinephrine levels in adults with ADHD, controlling the symptoms. bupropion (Wellbutrin) also shows promise in controlling ADHD symptoms by affecting the brain's dopamine levels.

- Psychotherapy and Education

    Adults with ADHD work with a professional therapist or counselor to learn to cope with ADHD. Learning how to organize is important. Tools like reminder notes, to-do lists or large calendars can help.

    Cognitive behavioral therapy helps in promoting a more positive self-image by helping the person examine the experiences that led to having a poor self-image.

Chapter 6 Parenting a Child With ADHD

Parents play a major role in helping children with ADHD. These children need the understanding and guidance of their parents, including teachers and other adults around them, in order for them to reach their full potential. Prior to diagnosis, families of children with ADHD may have dealt with anger, guilt, blame, and frustration over the child's condition. Family members should be given assistance in overcoming the negative feelings, in order for them to be better at handling the stress of raising a child with ADHD. Educate the family on what ADHD is, the symptoms, the treatments and how to effectively deal with the associated behaviors.

Some of the common situations where problems may arise include:

- getting your child to sleep at night
- arriving at school on time
- listening to and carrying out instructions
- social occasions
- shopping

To effectively deal and prevent problems, follow these guidelines:

- Rewards systems and consequences

  Parents should learn how to institute a system of rewards and consequences when dealing with a child's behavior. Give immediate feedback on certain behaviors. Do not wait for some time to pass, because chances are, the child already forgot the behavior and the events that lead to that specific conduct. Positive feedback is given to reinforce good behaviors and to encourage more of the desirable behavior in the future. Undesirable behaviors are ignored because even negative reactions are still attention that can reinforce a behavior. Redirect unruly behavior. If it gets out of control, use time-outs. Remove the child from the upsetting or stimulating situation and place him to a quiet room or corner. Stay with the child but do not try to talk, reason, and worse, argue with the child. Give him time to calm down.

- Share positive, pleasant, relaxing activities with the child.

This will help the parents to recognize more of the child's abilities rather than putting more focus on the negative aspect of ADHD symptoms. Parents should also take this opportunity to notice and praise the child for what he can achieve. This is also an opportunity for parents to recognize how to structure situations to help reduce the triggers of undesirable behaviors. Playmates may be limited to one to avoid overstimulation during playtime. Spending time with the child can also help parents know what tasks are too large for them to handle alone so that they can be able to divide the tasks into smaller ones.

- Create a schedule

Children with ADHD learn to be organized and complete tasks when a routine is followed. It also reduces the stimulation that immediate changes in activities bring.

Follow the same routine every day, from the time the child wakes up until bedtime. Schedule all activities like taking a bath, eating meals, doing homework, indoor activities like painting, outdoor play like time in the sandbox, naps and snacks.

Bedtime rituals should also be followed every night. Brushing the teeth, washing up, changing into bedclothes, massages, bedtime stories, even the lights-out routine should all be the same each night. This will help in dealing with sleeping problems due to the medication or too much excess energy. Poor or inadequate sleep creates a vicious cycle. The child wakes up too stressed, making him irritable all day long. By the next bedtime, problems will again arise, creating the same pattern the next day.

Should there be any changes, like the need to travel, prepare the child in advance. Introduce the idea of a change in schedule days before it happens. Allow the child to get used to the idea of changing an activity before instituting the change. This way, stress and frustration is reduced, and the child is less likely to act up.

- Organize the child's things

Keep specific items in their own specific place. Backpacks are to be placed in the same corner every time. Toys are put back in the same toy bin. Clothes are hung on a specific peg. These things not only help the child learn how to organize, it also reduces frustrations when the specific item cannot be found.

Homework and notebook organizers help the child to finish tasks. Stress the importance of writing down what needs to be done and to bring home the necessary materials for these tasks.

- Be clear and consistent with established rules

When a child acts out of line, reinforce the rules. Do not reprimand or give negative comments. They expect criticisms and ridicule from a lifetime of experience. Repeat the rules and the expected conduct. Give immediate and appropriate praise for good or positive behavior.

- Give clear and concise instructions

Children with ADHD are easily overwhelmed with large tasks and complicated instructions. Break down what needs to be done in small easy steps. Be clear on how a task is to be done and what the expected results are.

Instead of giving general instructions like "clean the room", be specific. Tell the child to "Put the green ball back to the blue toy box." Instead of telling the child to finish homework, specifically tell the child to finish the Math assignment on pages 15-17 of his workbook.

- Praise good behavior.

ADHD children are difficult. And dealing with them can be frustrating. But they do have their moments. It is important you pay attention. Use praise as a tool for disciplining the child. Use praises that are specific. Do not just say, "Excellent job." If the child correctly followed previous instructions, state the specific reason why he is getting praised. For instance, say something like "Excellent job for remembering to put your plate in the sink when you're finished just like I asked you."

Notice good behavior. Be kind and generous with praises. Praise the child for playing quietly, for following instructions and for sitting still.

- Teach the child Time-Out.

    This does not have to seem like just another form of punishment but as a way to calm down when he is angered or to keep it down a notch when he is feeling over-stimulated. Emphasize it is not a punishment but a strategy. It is a skill that the kid can develop and it can be an effective work around tool for ADHD. It can also be applied to different situations too. Make the child choose a quiet space where he can find calm and peace.

- Ignore slight misbehaviors.

    ADHD children are known for being attention seekers. This is why it is important to spend positive time with the child. If he gets enough attention, he may not resort to doing things in an effort to attract attention. Alternatively, you can simply ignore these mild misbehaviors.

    You do not have to notice every little action. If you are quite sure the child is misbehaving just to get some attention, resist. When the kid starts to whine, make loud noises, interrupt conversations or complain, ignore him. When you pay attention it only works to reinforce the behavior. When the child figures out he can get your attention by misbehaving slightly, he is more likely to stick to this strategy. So if it is a mild misbehavior, let it pass.

- Home and School Partnership

  As a parent, it is important to help your child work it out in all aspects of his life. But the school also plays a major role. With home and school working hand in hand, the child can have an increased chance of succeeding academically. Work it out with your child's teachers. With their help, create a better behavior management plan.

  Certain modifications may be necessary. For instance, it would not be too much to ask the teacher to give your child additional time to finish tests. If it will help the child to complete work and focus more if placed in a quieter and smaller environment then such can be arranged. The reward system you enforce at home may also be used by the teacher as strategy to help reinforce good behavior in the child.

ADHD and Anger in Children

One of the more challenging issues that with children who have ADHD is anger. Reacting with anger is quite common. And it is your job to help the child manage such emotions. In addition to anger, children with ADHD may also be hypersensitive. When they are faced with frustrating and stressful situations, they may response with intense anger.

In addition to managing the emotions, children with ADHD also find it challenging to think their problems through before reacting. Understand that you may not be able to help the child eliminate anger altogether. However, you can help him manage intense reactions better so he does not have to lose control.

So how do you exactly teach anger management to a kid? Below are a few suggestions.

- Get to know the triggers.

  You may have witnessed plenty of meltdowns and at this point, you should already have pinpointed common situations or matters that upset the child so leading to intense fits of anger. Take note of these instances.

  Is there a particular time during the day when your child seems to be angrier than usual? Is there a peak time? Do you see any patterns?

  ADHD children do not respond to school like most kids do. After school, he may feel tired or hungry. The problem is he may not be able to find a way to release whatever he is bottled up inside. Ask again, does your child get frustrated with specific tasks either for school or at home?

  When the medication starts to wear off, it could be a difficult time too. The bottom line is to take note of these triggers so you know the best way to catch an angry meltdown before it happens.

- Intervene as early as possible.

  Being aware of your child's anger triggers allows you to intervene quickly and early. Your presence should serve as a calming one. If your kid responds to physical contact, use it to calm him down. You can rub his arm or his back. Teach your child some breathing techniques. Encourage him to count to 10 while breathing deeply. And to be more effective, do it with him. It can help him release pent-up emotions.

- Teach him the value of time out.

Help your child realize that he does not have to respond to frustrating situations negatively. He can take time and cool down. But it can be challenging to teach him a time out skill during an anger fit. So, choose a time when your child is in a perfect mood and perfectly calm. At this time, he is most responsive to suggestion.

Talk with the kid about time-out and how he can use it. You can also turn this into a routine especially when you know his anger peak time is drawing near. Let him pick the spot. It could be a corner away from the craziness of the household. Make sure he understands how he can use time out when he is need of it.

When he does it, you can also guide him further by walking with him to the time out spot. Breathing exercises during a time out may help further. So do this with him. What you must avoid is to make an attempt to talk to him while he is angry. Wait it out until he is settled and completely calm. Praise him for being able to use time out effectively.

You can also encourage him to talk about what just happened. If he broke anything during his anger fit, help him understand there are other more productive ways of expressing his feelings. Suggest less harmful ways of releasing his emotions. And while you are talking to him, stay as calm as possible.

- Put labels to feelings.

When you notice that your child starts to get frustrated with a task, teach your kid how to reflect upon it too. You can start by saying, "This homework is a little difficult. And I can see that you are getting a little frustrated about it." These simple statements can enforce awareness. As your child becomes aware of his feelings, he learns to label them too.

When he comes home from school and you get a call from his teacher about having a rough time with his peers, sit him down. Talk to him about the way he felt in that situation. This will encourage him to use his own words in expressing his feelings.

- Suggest.

Do not just tell your child what to do. It is important you give him a sense of control. Offer choices. For instance, when he is having a rough time with a certain chore like cleaning up after himself, you can help him by saying, "Do you want to put the race cars away first or pick up the papers?" Limit the choices. When you offer too many, he can get a little overwhelmed and that can possibly lead to over-stimulation. So, it may be wiser to limit your suggestions to three.

- Make sure your child gets enough rest.

  Another problem ADHD kids experience is trouble with sleep. When someone does not get enough rest as they should, irritability sets in. When your child does not get enough sleep during the night, he will have more difficulty dealing with stress. He becomes moody and easily frustrated. Help him by figuring out strategies that can improve the quality of his sleep. This way, he can better handle the stresses during the day.

- Show him good anger management skills.

  How can you teach your child anger management skills when you also have trouble controlling yours? Teach him by example. Make it a point to respond to situations appropriately. Talk about the process with your child. Help him better understand it. Show him positive ways to respond to stressful situations better.

Adults may have ADHD, too. Signs include a history of failures in school, problems dealing with situations at work and difficulty maintaining relationships. They may also have a history of breaking the rules or laws like traffic violations. They are likely to engage in several activities at the same time, being all over the place, most of them unsuccessful endeavors. Adults with ADHD prefer doing quick fixes rather than go through all the steps to achieve a lasting and more rewarding result.

Chapter 7 Living with an Adult with ADHD

Roughly four percent of US adults have ADHD. Adults who have not been diagnosed with ADHD as a child and have never received treatment or medication of any kind. Early diagnosis and intervention are essential in these situations. Adults with ADHD who have received appropriate treatment since childhood cope much better than those who just received treatment later on.

In any case, adults also need to learn how to deal with their ADHD. Here are quick guides n how to exercise control over the symptoms.

- Stop impulses.

  This is a difficult task but it can be done. To start, be aware of situations that lead to impulsive behaviors. Make a list every time an impulse is felt and when it is acted out. This way, the person can review behaviors and be aware of what triggers them. When the person finds himself in the same situation, take a few seconds to think about the consequences. Recall the events in the past where in the same thing happened and recall the negative consequences of the actions.

  This helps in developing hindsight and foresight. These skills are helpful in dealing with impulses and preventing acting out the impulsive behaviors. Some tips include:

  - Inhaling an exhaling slowly, think hard about the responses, how it should be expressed and the possible consequences of these responses.

- o Should an impulse to answer someone occurs, place a finger over the mouth, put a thoughtful expression and tell the other person to give you time to think over what has been said to you.

- o Paraphrase what has been said to clarify the intent and to help in providing more time to organize thoughts and words.

- o Consciously slow down when talking. Instead of talking a 100-words per minute, speak words slowly, as if trying to put emphasis on every spoken word. This way, you avoid blabbering and saying things you might regret later.

- Learn from the past and move on

Mistakes happen. Awkward situations occur. Learn to forgive yourself and let go of the mistakes. Look for the lessons in those situations and make it a point to not let it happen again in the future.

Take the opportunity of mistakes as a learning tool. Most adults affected with ADHD cannot see the subtleties and differences of problems. To them, all problems are the same and react in the same way. Mistakes are opportunities to recognize the differences in situations that lead to problems, mistakes, arguments or other negative consequences.

- Keep an eye on the future

Most adults fail to complete tasks because they easily forget the rewards. They lose track of the goals they have set. Start learning memory recall. Learn to view what was the purpose, the goal. For example, keep envisioning a large flat screen TV as a reward after finishing a project at work. The more often the vision is recalled, the more it will stick to the mind, the more motivated the person will be to complete the task.

- Break it down

As with children, adults suffering from ADHD can be easily overwhelmed with large tasks. They also have trouble following complex instructions. People with ADHD may call in sick when the going gets tough. They may resort to behaviors like indifference or lack of enthusiasm mainly because they became overwhelmed or frustrated with the enormity of a task.

To cope with this difficulty, break down a large task into smaller ones. The mist helpful is to make the smaller tasks yield more meaningful results. These small but meaningful results are great incentives and keep the person motivated to continue with the other small tasks, until eventually the larger result is achieved.

Example is to break each required step into hourly goals. Schedule the first hour of the morning as the time to gather the materials for the task. The second hour is dedicated to organizing these materials. The third is for a break and assess what has been done and what still needs to be accomplished, and so on.

After each mini-task is completed, congratulate the self, make a big check mark on the to-do list and take a short break.

Chapter 8 How to Help Yourself Help Someone with ADHD

Knowing that a dear loved one has ADHD can push you through a mixture of strange feelings. ADHD is difficult for the sufferer. But it also takes a toll on the people around. The key to making life easier is to educate yourself. If you want to help someone cope with ADHD, you have to start by gaining a much better understanding about the disorder. With this said, here are a few suggestions.

Read.

There are plenty of online references and books that can help educate you about ADHD. In addition to reading, make sure to ask questions from the doctor. To figure out strategies, you can also talk with parents or other families dealing with ADHD.

Get support.

When your child has ADHD, you and your spouse should always be on the same page when it comes to parenting. You have to be consistent and united with disciplining techniques. Parenting a child with ADHD can be physically exhausting and emotionally draining. This means each parent may need some time and space alone, a break for parenting. Give each other that.

The situation can be a little more challenging for single parents. If you are one, get support from your family. Hire a babysitter and make sure you choose a trusted one. Orient the babysitter about your strategies to build consistency.

Join family therapy.

There are parenting programs that are designed to help you figure out the most appropriate parenting strategies. There are behavioral specialists who can help you create a behavioral program specific to your situation. It can indeed be quite helpful.

Acting as one unit is important and since ADHD can affect the entire family, joining therapy can also help you sort out issues. It is not only helpful for the people around the patient. But it is extremely beneficial to the person with ADHD too. This way, the patient gets all the support he needs.

Laugh.

Laughter is the best medicine as they say. It provides a great relief during stressful situations. Humor is a great way of dealing with frustration.

Conclusion

Thank you again for purchasing this book!

I hope this book was able to help you to understand what ADHD is all about. It is not something that should hinder anyone from living a full life. It can be dealt with, given the right information, understanding and guides on dealing with the problems that arise.

The next step is to start making a conscious effort to help someone, or yourself, deal with ADHD.

Finally, if you enjoyed this book, please take the time to share your thoughts and post a review on Amazon. We do our best to reach out to readers and provide the best value we can. Your positive review will help us achieve that. It'd be greatly appreciated!

Thank you and good luck!

Check Out My Other Books

Below you'll find some of my other popular books that are popular on Amazon and Kindle as well. Simply click on the links below to check them out. Alternatively, you can visit my author page on Amazon to see other work done by me.

Cure For Controlling People: The Ultimate Guide for Releasing You from Those That Control You In A Relationship

http://www.amazon.com/Cure-Controlling-People-Relationship-Codependency-ebook/dp/B00JOHTV5K

ADHD Symptom and Strategies: The Ultimate Guide for Understanding and Handling Attention Deficit Disorder in Adults and Children

http://www.amazon.com/ADHD-Symptom-Strategies-Understanding-Hyperactivity-ebook/dp/B00JOZT3DM

Narcissism Unleashed 2nd Edition! The Ultimate Guide to Understanding the Mind of a Narcissist, Sociopath and Psychopath!

http://www.amazon.com/Narcissism-Understanding-Narcissist-Narcissistic-Personality-ebook/dp/B00JP0UQM8

How to Cure the Workaholic Addiction: Control Anxiety and Stress Before It's Too Late!

http://www.amazon.com/How-Cure-Workaholic-Addiction-Workaholics-ebook/dp/B00JPZJY2Q/

Living with Autism: The Successful Steps to Recognizing, Adapting, Learning, and Understanding Autism

http://www.amazon.com/Living-Autism-Recognizing-Understanding-Breakthrough-ebook/dp/B00JQS6Z5Q

The Ultimate Self Esteem Guide: Steps to Building Self Esteem, Confidence, and Inner strength!

http://www.amazon.com/Ultimate-Self-Esteem-Guide-Codependancy-ebook/dp/B00JY2F3K2

The Shopping Addiction: A Cure for Compulsive Shopping and Spending to Free Yourself from Addiction!

http://www.amazon.com/Shopping-Addiction-Compulsive-Self-Help-Impulsive-ebook/dp/B00JY2FYDS

Living With OCD: A Powerful Guide To Understanding Obsessive Compulsive Disorder In Children And Adults

http://www.amazon.com/Living-OCD-Understanding-Compulsive-Personality-ebook/dp/B00K3E3E06

BOX SET #1: Narcissism Unleashed! & Cure For Controlling People

http://www.amazon.com/BOX-SET-Controlling-Narcissistic-Codependency-ebook/dp/B00KAATSFI

BOX SET #2: Narcissism Unleashed! & Mind Control Mastery

http://www.amazon.com/BOX-SET-Narcissistic-Personality-Manifestation-ebook/dp/B00K9URU90

BOX SET #3 ADHD Symptoms & Strategies & Living With OCD

http://www.amazon.com/Symptoms-Strategies-Attention-attention-hyperactivity-ebook/dp/B00KA0K4SI

BOX SET #4: Living With OCD & The Ultimate Self Esteem Guide

http://www.amazon.com/BOX-SET-Ultimate-Confidence-Strength-ebook/dp/B00KA0U04G

BOX SET #5: Narcissism Unleashed! & Mind Control Mastery & The Shopping Addiction & Living With OCD & The Ultimate Self Esteem Guide

http://www.amazon.com/Box-Set-Narcissism-Compulsive-Psychopath-ebook/dp/B00KK96T56

If the links do not work, for whatever reason, you can simply search for these titles on the Amazon website to find them.